The Best Pressure Cooker Fish Recipes

Easy and Tasty Recipes for Pressure Cooker

Cheryl J. Pickett

Sommario

Introduction

The Ninja Foodi multi-cooker is one of the devices that every person ought to have in their kitchen area. The device can change four little tools: sluggish cooker, air fryer, pressure cooker and dehydrator.

This recipe book includes a few of the dishes we have actually tried with the multi-cooker. The recipes vary from morning meal, side dishes, poultry, pork, soups, fish and shellfish, desserts, and also pasta. In addition, we have actually compiled lots of vegan dishes you ought to try. We developed these dishes considering novices which's why the cooking procedure is methodical. Besides, the dishes are tasty, take pleasure in reading.

FISH AND SEAFOOD

Tuna Patties

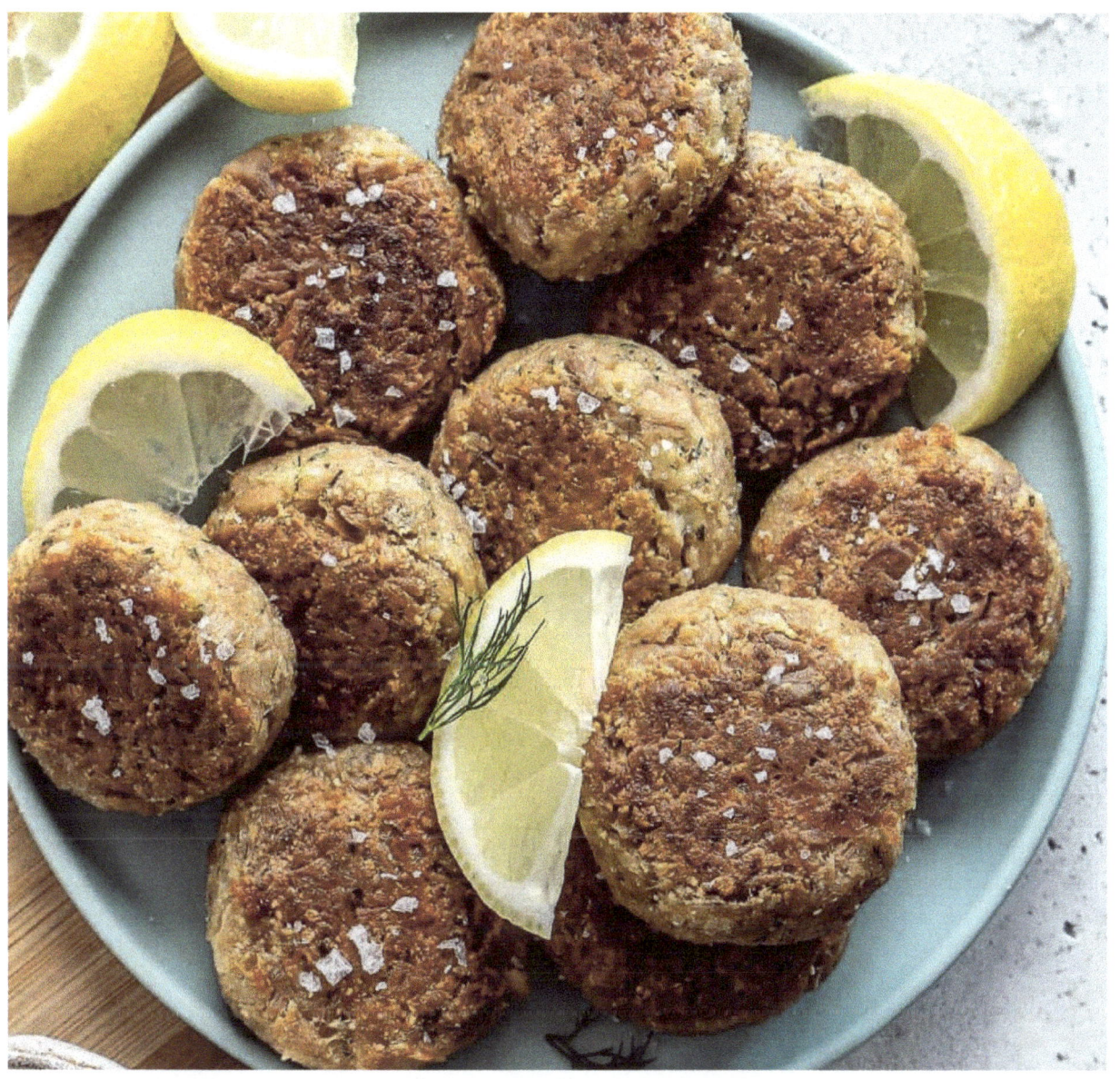

INGREDIENTS (2 Servings)

2 cans tuna flakes

1/2 tablespoon almond flour

1 teaspoon dried dill 1 tablespoon mayo

1/2 teaspoon onion powder

1 teaspoon garlic powder

Salt and pepper to taste

1 tablespoon lemon juice

DIRECTIONS (PREP + COOK TIME: 30 MINUTES)

 Mix all the ingredients in a bowl. Form patties. Set the tuna patties on the Ninja Foodi basket. Seal the crisping lid. Set it to air crisp. Cook at 400 degrees for 10 minutes. Flip and cook for 5 more minutes. Serving

Crispy Cod Fish

INGREDIENTS (4 Servings)

4 cod fish fillets

Salt and sugar to taste

1 teaspoon sesame oil

250 ml water

5 tablespoons light soy sauce

1 teaspoon dark soy sauce

3 tablespoons oil

5 slices ginger

DIRECTIONS (PREP + COOK TIME: 30 MINUTES)

Pat the cod fish fillets dry. Season with the salt, sugar and sesame oil. Marinate for 15 minutes. Set the Ninja Foodi to air crisp. Put the fish on top of the basket. Cook at 350 degrees F for 3 minutes. Flip and cook for 2 minutes. Take the fish out and set aside. Put the rest of the ingredients in the pot. Set it to sauté. Simmer and pour over the fish before serving. Serving

Heartfelt Sesame Fish

INGREDIENTS (4 Servings)

1 and ½ pound salmon fillet

1 teaspoon sesame seeds

1 teaspoon butter, melted

½ teaspoon salt

1 tablespoon apple cider vinegar

¼ teaspoon rosemary, dried

DIRECTIONS (PREP + COOK TIME: 16 MINUTES)

Take apple cider vinegar and spray it to the salmon fillets Then add dried rosemary, sesame seeds, butter and salt Mix them well.

Take butter sauce and brush the salmon properly Place the salmon on the rack and lower the air fryer lid. Set the air fryer mode Cook the fish for 8 minutes at 360 F.Serve hot and enjoy!

Buttered Up Scallops

INGREDIENTS (4 Servings)

4 garlic cloves, minced

4 tablespoons rosemary, chopped

2 pounds sea scallops

12 cup butter

Salt and pepper to taste

DIRECTIONS (PREP + COOK TIME: 15 MINUTES)

Set your Ninja Foodi to Saute mode and add butter, rosemary, and garlic Saute for 1 minute. Add scallops, salt, and pepper Saute for 2 minutes. Lock Crisping lid and Crisp for 3 minutes at 350 degrees F. Serve and enjoy!

Lovely Air Fried Scallops

INGREDIENTS (4 Servings)

12 scallops

3 tablespoons olive oil

Salt and pepper to taste

DIRECTIONS (PREP + COOK TIME: 10 MINUTES)

Gently rub scallops with salt, pepper, and oil Transfer to your Ninja Foodie's insert, and place the insert in your Foodi Lock Air Crisping lid and cook for 4 minutes at 390 degrees F Half through, make sure to give them a nice flip and keep cooking. Serve warm and enjoy!

Garlic And Lemon Prawn Delight

INGREDIENTS (4 Servings)

2 tablespoons olive oil

1 pound prawns

2 tablespoons garlic, minced

2/3 cup fish stock

1 tablespoon butter

2 tablespoons lemon juice

1 tablespoon lemon zest

Salt and pepper to taste

DIRECTIONS (PREP + COOK TIME: 10 MINUTES)

Set your Ninja Foodi to Saute mode and add butter and oil, let it heat up Stir in remaining ingredients. Lock lid and cook on LOW pressure for 5 minutes Quick release pressure. Serve and enjoy!

Lovely Panko Cod

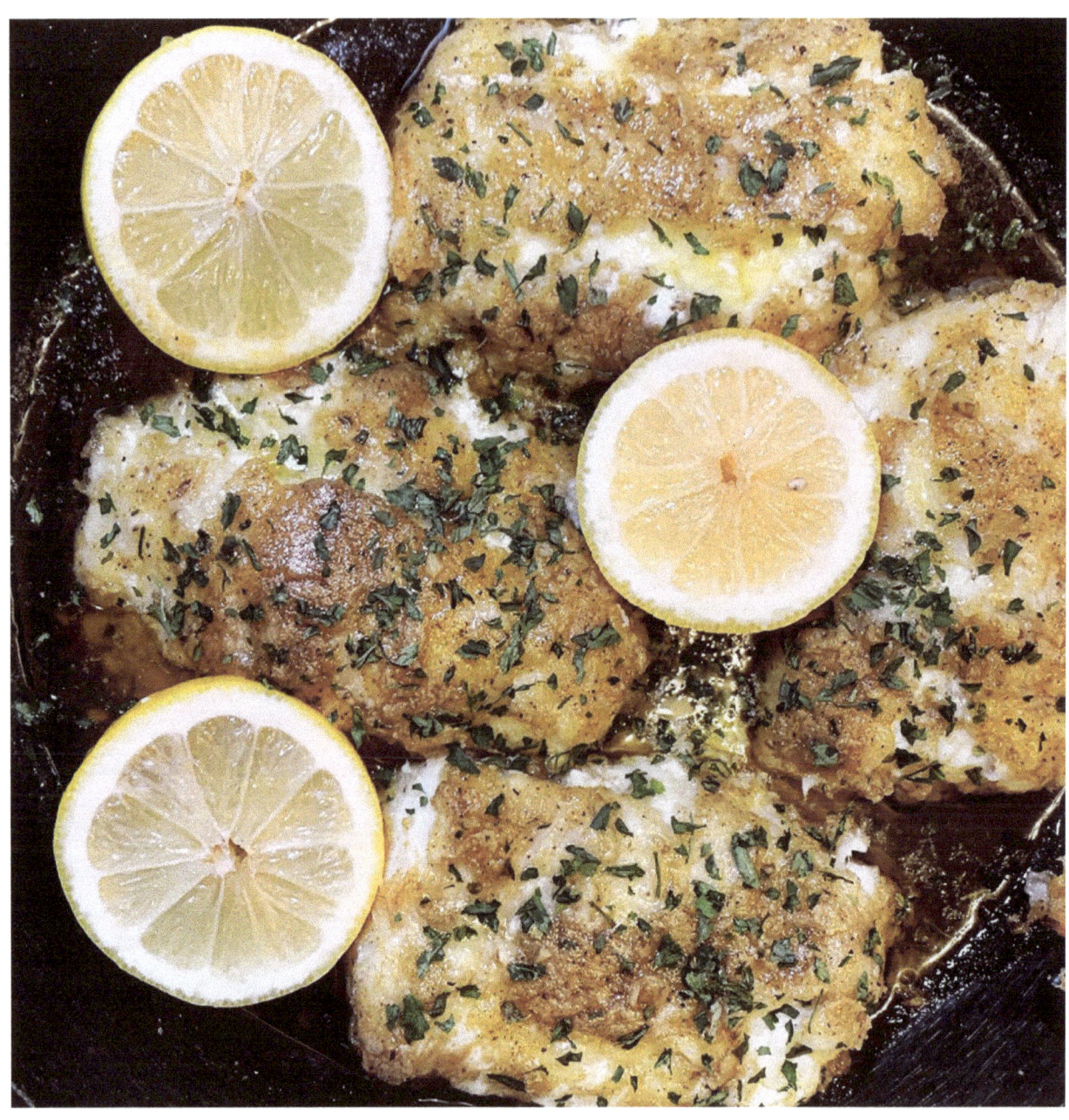

INGREDIENTS (6 Servings)

2 uncooked cod fillets,

6 ounces each

3 teaspoons kosher salt

¾ cup panko bread crumbs

2 tablespoons butter, melted

¼ cup fresh parsley, minced

1 lemon.

Zested and juiced

DIRECTIONS (PREP + COOK TIME: 20 MINUTES)

Pre-heat your Ninja Foodi at 390 degrees F and place Air Crisper basket inside Season cod and salt Take a bowl and add bread crumbs, parsley, lemon juice, zest, butter, and mix well Coat fillets with the bread crumbs mixture and place fillets in your Air Crisping basket Lock Air Crisping lid and cook on Air Crisp mode for 15 minutes at 360 degrees F Serve and enjoy!

Ranch Warm Fillets

INGREDIENTS (4 Servings)

¼ cup panko

½ packet ranch dressing mix powder

1 and ¼ tablespoons vegetable oil

1 egg beaten

2 tilapia fillets

A garnish of herbs and chilies

DIRECTIONS (PREP + COOK TIME: 18 MINUTES)

Pre-heat your Ninja Foodi with the Crisping Basket inside at 350 degrees F Take a bowl and mix in ranch dressing and panko Beat eggs in a shallow bowl and keep it on the side Dip fillets in the eggs, then in the panko mix Place fillets in your Ninja Foodie's insert and transfer insert to Ninja Foodi Lock Air Crisping Lid and Air Crisp for 13 minutes at 350 degrees F Garnish with chilies and herbs. Enjoy!

Kale And Salmon Delight

INGREDIENTS (4 Servings)

1 lemon, juiced

2 salmon fillets

¼ cup extra virgin olive oil

1 teaspoon Dijon mustard

4 cups kale, thinly sliced, ribs removed

1 teaspoon salt

1 avocado, diced

1 cup pomegranate seeds

1 cup walnuts, toasted

1 cup goat parmesan cheese, shredded

DIRECTIONS (PREP + COOK TIME: 15 MINUTES)

Season salmon with salt and keep it on the side. Place a trivet in your Ninja Foodi Place salmon over the trivet. Lock lid and cook on HIGH pressure for 15 minutes Release pressure naturally over 10 minutes. Transfer salmon to a serving platter Take a bowl and add kale, season with salt Take another bowl and make the dressing by adding lemon juice, Dijon mustard, olive oil, and red wine vinegar. Season kale with dressing and add diced avocado, pomegranate seeds, walnuts and cheese. Toss and serve with the fish. Enjoy!

Lemon And Pepper Salmon Delight

INGREDIENTS (4 Servings)

¾ cup of water

Sprigs of parsley, basil, tarragon

1 pound salmon, skin on

3 teaspoons ghee

¾ teaspoon salt

½ teaspoon pepper

 ½ lemon, sliced

1 red bell pepper, julienned

1 carrot, julienned

DIRECTIONS (PREP + COOK TIME: 11 MINUTES)

Set your Ninja Foodi to Saute mode and add water and herbs Place a steamer rack and add the salmon. Drizzle ghee on top of the salmon Season with pepper and salt. Cover lemon slices on top Lock up the lid and cook on HIGH pressure for 3 minutes Release the pressure naturally over 10 minutes Transfer the salmon to a platter. Add veggies to your pot and set the pot to Saute mode Cook for 1-2 minutes. Serve the cooked vegetables with salmon. Enjoy!

Ranch Fish Fillet

INGREDIENTS (4 Servings)

3/4 cup bread crumbs

1 packet dry ranch dressing mix 2

1/2 tablespoons vegetable oil

2 eggs, beaten 4 fish fillets

DIRECTIONS (PREP + COOK TIME: 20 MINUTES)

Combine the bread crumbs and ranch mix in a bowl. Pour in the oil. Dip each fish fillet into the egg and cover with the crumb mixture. Place in the Ninja Foodi basket. Seal the lid. Select air crisp function.Cook at 360 degrees F for 12 minutes, flipping halfway through. Serving

Paprika Salmon

INGREDIENTS (2 Servings)

2 salmon fillets

2 teaspoons avocado oil

2 teaspoons paprika

Salt and pepper to taste

DIRECTIONS (PREP + COOK TIME: 15 MINUTES)

Coat the salmon with oil. Season with salt, pepper and paprika. Place in the Ninja Foodi basket. Set it to air crisp function. Seal the crisping lid. Cook at 390 degrees for 7 minutes. Serving

Southern Fried Fish Fillet

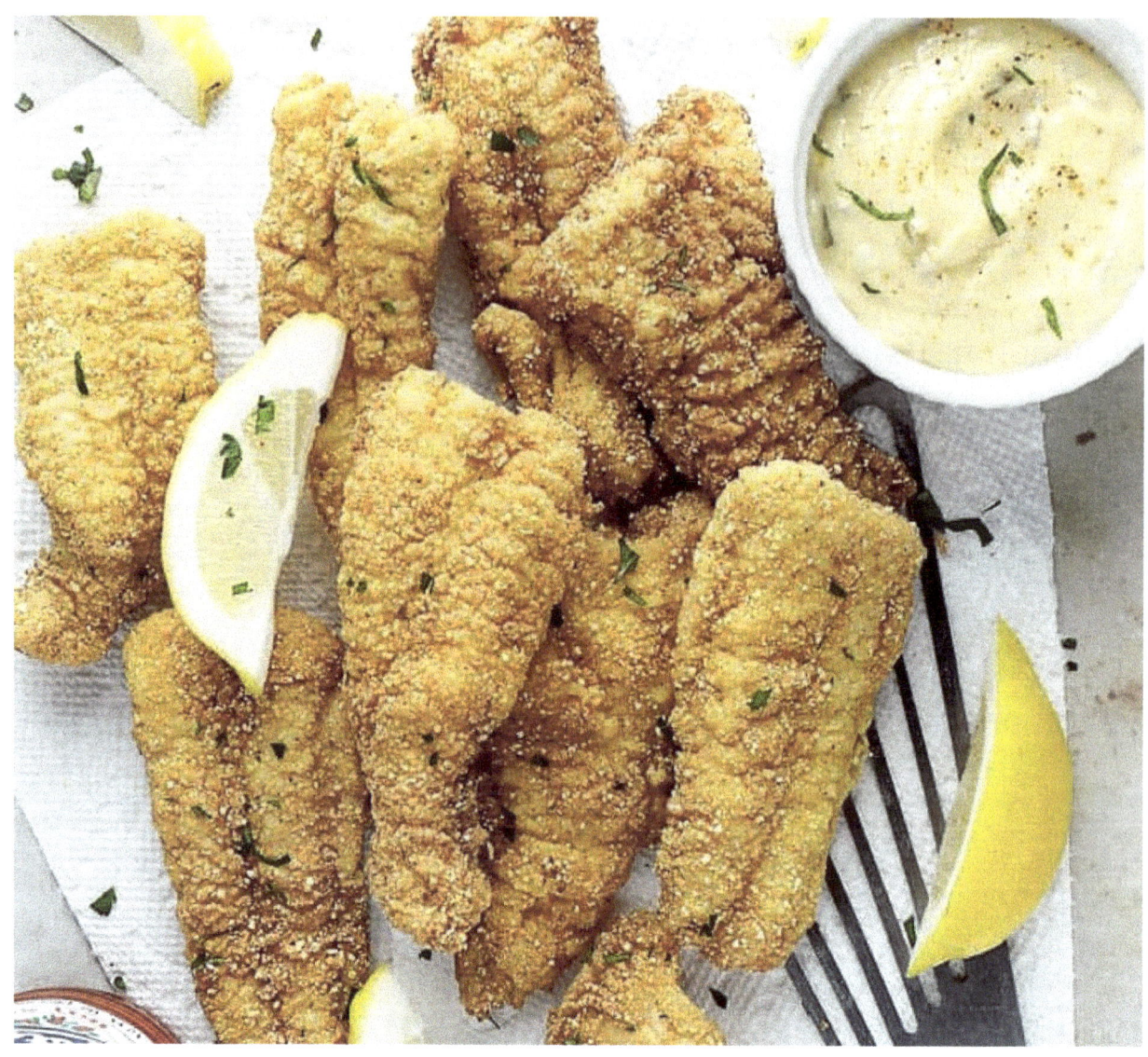

INGREDIENTS (4 Servings)

2 lb. white fish fillet

1 cup low fat milk

1 lemon slice

1/2 cup mustard

1/2 cup cornmeal

1/4 cup all purpose flour

2 tablespoons dried parsley flakes

Salt and pepper to taste

1/4 teaspoon chili powder

1/4 teaspoon garlic powder

1/4 teaspoon onion powder

1/4 teaspoon cayenne pepper

DIRECTIONS (PREP + COOK TIME: 30 MINUTES)

Place the fish fillet in a bowl. Pour the milk over the fish fillet. Squeeze lemon slice over the fish. Marinate for 15 minutes. Spread the mustard on the fish fillets. In another bowl, mix the rest of the ingredients. Coat the fish fillets with the cornmeal mixture. Place on the Ninja Foodi basket. Set it to air crisp. Seal the crisping lid. Cook at 390 degrees for 10 minutes.Flip the fillets and cook for 5 more minutes. Serving

Fish Fillet with Pesto Sauce

INGREDIENTS (3 Servings)

3 white fish fillets

1 tablespoon olive oil

Salt and pepper to taste

2 cups fresh basil leaves

 2 cloves garlic, crushed

2 tablespoons pine nuts

1 tablespoon Parmesan cheese, grated

1 cup olive oil

DIRECTIONS (PREP + COOK TIME: 20 MINUTES)

Coat the fish fillets with 1 tablespoon of olive oil. Season with the salt and pepper. Place in the Ninja Foodi basket. Cook at 320 degrees for 8 minutes. While waiting, mix the remaining ingredients in a food processor. Pulse until smooth. Spread the pesto sauce on both sides of the fish before serving. Serving

Coconut Shrimp

INGREDIENTS (4 Servings)

1/2 cup all purpose flour

1 1/2 teaspoons black pepper

2 eggs

1/3 cup panko bread crumbs

2/3 cup unsweetened coconut flakes

12 oz. shrimp, peeled and deveined

Cooking spray

Salt and pepper to taste

1/4 cup honey

1/4 cup lime juice

DIRECTIONS (PREP + COOK TIME: 20 MINUTES)

Mix the flour and black pepper in a bowl. In another bowl, beat the egg. In the third bowl, mix the bread crumbs and coconut flakes. Dip each of the shrimp in the first, second and third bowls. Place in the Ninja Foodi basket. Set it to air crisp.Cover the crisping lid. Cook at 400 degrees F for 8 minutes, turn halfway through. Season with the salt and pepper. Mix the remaining ingredients and serve with the shrimp. Serving

Crispy Shrimp

INGREDIENTS (4 Servings)

1 lb. shrimp, peeled and deveined

2 eggs

1/2 cup bread crumbs

1/2 cup onion, diced

1 teaspoon ginger

1 teaspoon garlic powder

Salt and pepper to taste

DIRECTIONS (PREP + COOK TIME: 20 MINUTES)

In one bowl, beat the two eggs. In another bowl, put the rest of the ingredients.Dip the shrimp first in the eggs and then in the spice mixture. Place in the Ninja Foodi basket.Seal the crisping lid. Choose air crisp function. Cook at 350 degrees for 10 minutes. Serving

Salt and Pepper Shrimp

INGREDIENTS (4 Servings)

2 teaspoons peppercorns

1 teaspoon salt

1 teaspoons sugar

1 lb. shrimp

3 tablespoons rice flour

2 tablespoons oil

DIRECTIONS (PREP + COOK TIME: 20 MINUTES)

Set the Ninja Foodi to sauté. Roast the peppercorns for 1 minute. Let them cool. Crush the peppercorns and add the salt and sugar. Coat the shrimp with this mixture and then with flour. Sprinkle oil on the Ninja Foodi basket. Place the shrimp on top. Cook at 350 degrees for 10 minutes, flipping halfway through. Serving

Lemon Garlic Shrimp

INGREDIENTS (4 Servings)

1 lb. shrimp, peeled and deveined

1 tablespoon olive oil

4 cloves garlic, minced

1 tablespoon lemon juice

Salt to taste

DIRECTIONS (PREP + COOK TIME: 40 MINUTES)

Mix the olive oil, salt, lemon juice and garlic.Toss shrimp in the mixture. Marinate for 15 minutes. Place the shrimp in the Ninja Foodi basket. Seal the crisping lid. Select the air crisp setting. Cook at 350 degrees for 8 minutes. Flip and cook for 2 more minutes. Serving

Crispy Fish Nuggets

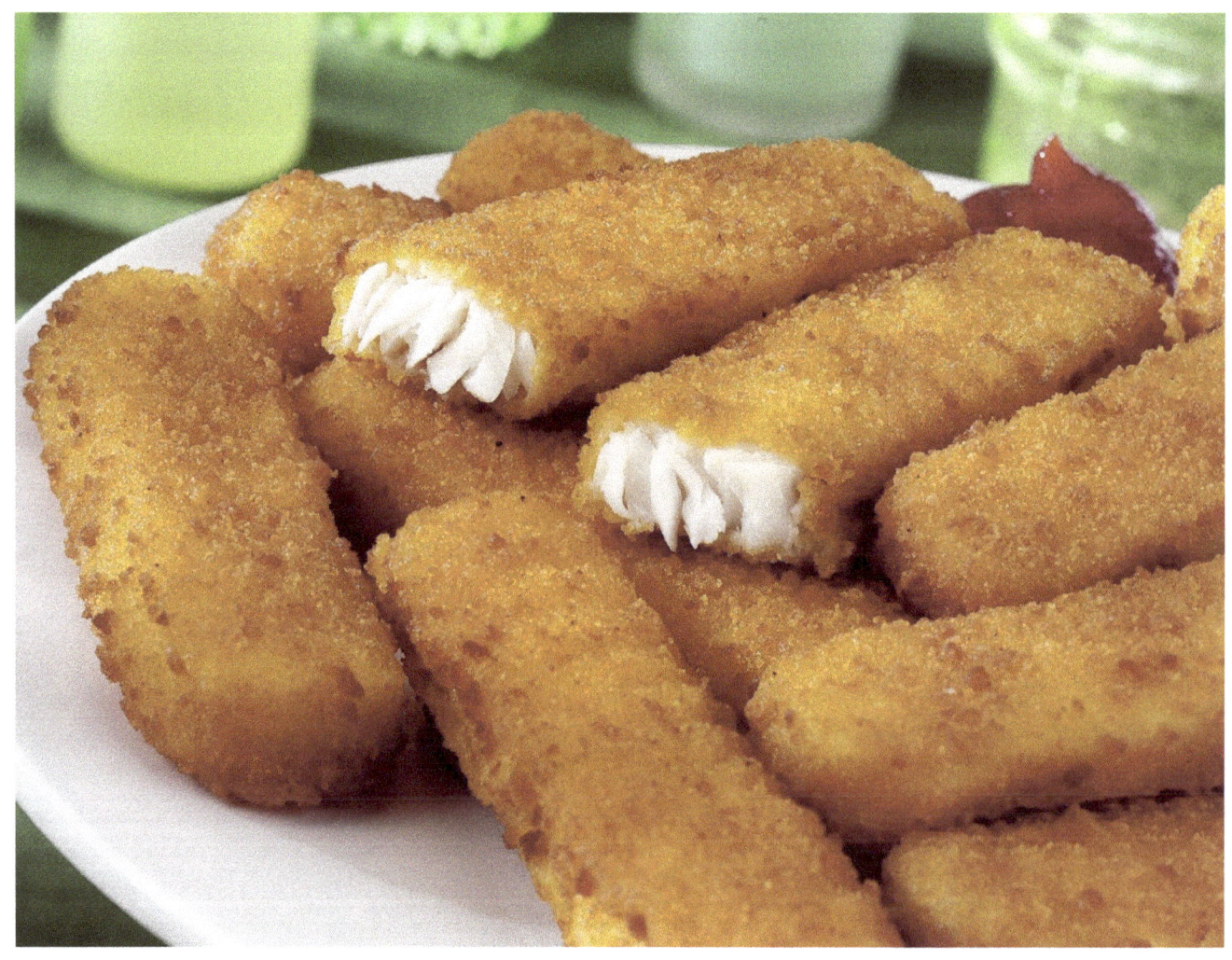

INGREDIENTS (4 Servings)

1 lb. cod fillet, sliced into

8 pieces Salt and pepper to taste

1/2 cup flour

1 tablespoon egg with

1 teaspoon water

1 cup bread crumbs

1 tablespoon vegetable oil

DIRECTIONS (PREP + COOK TIME: 30 MINUTES)

Season the fish with salt and pepper. Cover with the flour. Dip the fish in the egg wash and into the bread crumbs. Place the fish nuggets in the Ninja Foodi basket. Set it to air crisp function. Seal with the crisping lid. Cook at 360 degrees for 15 minutes. Serving

Awesome Sock-Eye Salmon

INGREDIENTS (4 Servings)

4 sockeye salmon fillets

1 teaspoon Dijon mustard

¼ teaspoon garlic, minced

¼ teaspoon onion powder

¼ teaspoon lemon pepper

½ teaspoon garlic powder

¼ teaspoon salt

2 tablespoons olive oil

1 and ½ cup of water

DIRECTIONS (PREP + COOK TIME: 10 MINUTES)

Take a bowl and add mustard, lemon juice, onion powder, lemon pepper, garlic powder, salt, olive oil. Brush spice mix over salmon Add water to Instant Pot. Place rack and place salmon fillets on rack Lock lid and cook on LOW pressure for 7 minutes Quick release pressure .Serve and enjoy!

Awesome Cherry Tomato Mackerel

INGREDIENTS (4 Servings)

4 Mackerel fillets

¼ teaspoon onion powder

¼ teaspoon lemon powder

¼ teaspoon garlic powder

½ teaspoon salt

2 cups cherry tomatoes

3 tablespoons melted butter

1 and ½ cups of water

1 tablespoon black olives

DIRECTIONS (PREP + COOK TIME: 12 MINUTES)

Grease baking dish and arrange cherry tomatoes at the bottom of the dish Top with fillets sprinkle all spices. Drizzle melted butter over Add water to your Ninja Foodi Lower rack in Ninja Foodi and place baking dish on top of the rack Lock lid and cook on LOW pressure for 7 minutes . Quick release pressure. Serve and enjoy!

Paella

INGREDIENTS (4-6 Servings)

2 tablespoons of extra virgin olive oil

3 links of chorizo, sliced

3 boneless skinless chicken thighs (cut)

1 medium onion (peeled and chopped finely)

2 cloves of garlic (peeled and minced)

 1 small red bell pepper, chopped

A teaspoon of paprika

1/2 teaspoon of oregano, dried

1/4 teaspoon of crushed red pepper

1/2 teaspoon of pepper

A teaspoon of kosher salt

Pinch of saffron threads, crumbled

A can (14 oz) of diced tomatoes

1/2 cup of chicken stock

1/4 cup of white wine

A cup of basmati rice

1 pound of mussels (scrubbed and de-bearded)

1 bag (12 oz) of frozen jumbo shrimp (peeled and deveined)

Juice from one lemon

2 tablespoons of fresh parsley, for garnishing

DIRECTIONS (PREP + COOK TIME: 27 MINUTES) Preheat your Foodi on sauté mode for a minute. Add the chicken thighs and sliced chorizos in oil. Cook for 5 minutes. Add the onions, garlic, red pepper, and spices. Sauté for another 5 minutes. Add the wine, stock, rice, tomatoes, shrimp, and mussels. Stir. Close the pressure lid and cook for 2 minutes. Quick release the accumulated pressure and open the lid. Transfer your Paella into a large bowl. Serve while topped with parsley and fresh lemon juice.

Seared Shrimp and Rice with Fruity

INGREDIENTS (4 Servings)

A cup of basmati rice

1 cup of water

1 1/2 teaspoons of sea salt, divided

3 tablespoons of canola oil

3 tablespoons of fresh lime juice, divided

1 lb (31-35) of large shrimp, uncooked

1 1/2 teaspoons of crab seasoning

A teaspoon of garlic powder

1 teaspoon of smoked paprika

1/2 teaspoon of onion powder

1 mango (peeled and chopped)

1/2 teaspoon of sugar

1/4 cup of red onion (peeled and chopped)

1 small bell pepper (red,) chopped

1/2 cup of pineapple, chopped

3 scallions, finely sliced 1 avocado, sliced

DIRECTIONS (PREP + COOK TIME: 30 MINUTES) Peel the shrimp, devein it and remove its tail. Put it aside. If frozen, thaw it first. Add, water, rice, and a teaspoon of salt in the Foodi. Close the pressure lid and cook on high mode for 2 minutes. Quick release the in-built pressure and open the lid. Meanwhile, toss the shrimp with the crab seasoning, onion powder, garlic powder, sugar, smoked paprika, and 2 tablespoons of oil. Open the pressure lid and add the remaining oil and a teaspoon of lime juice. Stir. Fix the rack in the rice-pot. Place shrimp on the rack and close the crisping lid. Broil it for 7 minutes. Halfway, open the lid and flip the shrimp. Meanwhile, add the mango, pineapple, bell pepper, red onion, the remaining salt and the lime juice. After the cooking time elapses, serve the broiled shrimp with rice. Top with avocado slices, scallions, and salsa.

Garlic Shrimp with Risotto Primavera

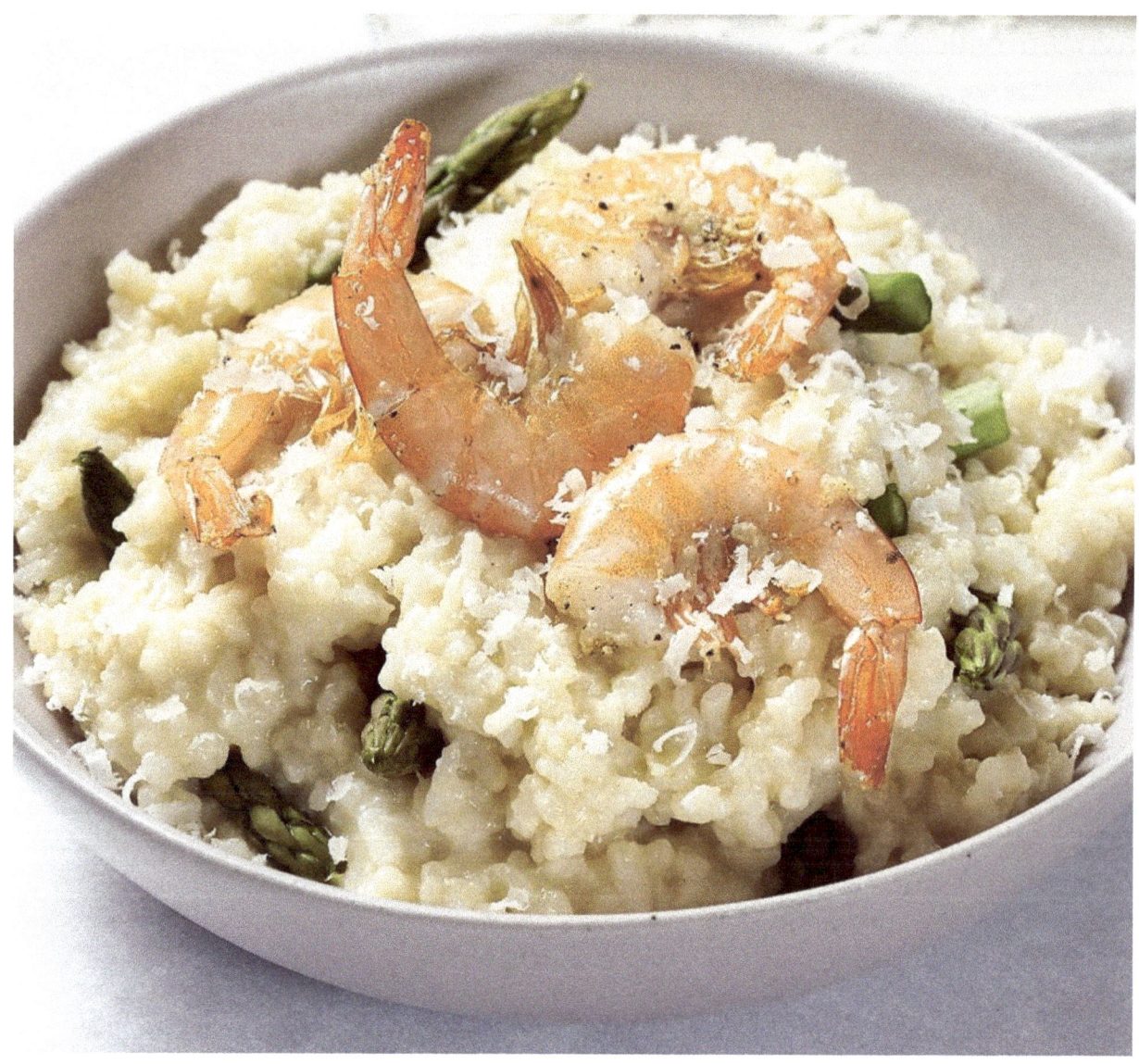

INGREDIENTS (4 Servings)

2 tablespoons of organic olive oil, divided

1 small onion (peeled and diced finely)

4 cloves garlic (peeled, minced, and divided)

3 teaspoons of sea salt, divided

5 1/2 cups of chicken stock

2 glasses of short- grained rice

16 uncooked jumbo shrimp (peeled and deveined)

2 teaspoons of garlic powder

1 teaspoon of ground black pepper

2 tablespoons of butter Juice from a lemon

1 bunch of asparagus (trimmed and cut)

1 1/2 cups of grated Parmesan cheese

DIRECTIONS (PREP + COOK TIME: 39 MINUTES) Set your Foodi to sauté mode. Add a tablespoon of oil. Add the onion and cook until it softens. Add half of the garlic and cook for 1 minute or until its fragrant. Add 2 teaspoons of salt, stock, and rice. Close the pressure lid. Toss the shrimp in the oil and add the remaining garlic, garlic powder, salt, and black pepper. Let the pressure release naturally for 10 minutes before quick releasing the rest. Open the lid and add butter, fresh lemon juice, and asparagus into it. Fix the reversible rack over the risotto and add the shrimp into the rack. Close the crisping lid and broil for 8 minutes. Remove the rack and add Parmesan into the risotto. Stir. Serve your meal while topped with shrimp and Parmesan.

Salmon with Orange Ginger Sauce

INGREDIENTS (4 Servings)

1 pound of salmon

2 teaspoons of minced ginger

1 tablespoon of dark soy sauce

1 teaspoon of garlic, minced

½ teaspoon of salt

1-11/2 teaspoon of ground pepper

2 tablespoons of marmalade, low sugar

DIRECTIONS (PREP + COOK TIME: 30 MINUTES) Put salmon in a Ziploc bag. Add the minced ginger, dark soy sauce, garlic, marmalade, salt, and pepper. Let it marinate for 30 minutes. Add 2 glasses of water in the Foodi. Fix a reversible rack over it and add the seasoned salmon with sauce. Close the pressure lid and cook on low mode for 3 minutes. Allow the in-built pressure to escape naturally. Close the crisping lid and broil the contents for 3 minutes. Alternatively, bake the seasoned fish at a temperature of 350°F for 5 minutes.

Thai Shrimp Soup Lime,

INGREDIENTS (6 Servings)

2 tablespoons of unsalted butter, divided

½ lb of medium shrimp (uncooked, peeled, and deveined)

½ yellow onion, diced

2 cloves of garlic, minced

2 tablespoons of fish sauce

4 servings of chicken broth

2 tablespoons of lime juice

1 tablespoon of coconut aminos or tamari sauce

2½ teaspoons of red curry paste

1 stalk of lemongrass (bruised and chopped)

1 cup of fresh white mushrooms, sliced

1 tablespoon of fresh cinnamon, grated

½ teaspoon of freshly ground black pepper

1 teaspoon of sea salt

1 can(13.66-oz) of unsweetened, full-fat coconut milk

3 tablespoons of fresh cilantro, chopped

DIRECTIONS (PREP + COOK TIME: 11 MINUTES) Set your Foodi to sauté mode. Add a tablespoon of butter and allow it to melt. Add the shrimp and stir until it turns pink. Transfer it into a bowl and set aside. Add the remaining butter into the pot and let it melt. Add onion and the garlic. Sauté for 3 minutes or until it turns translucent.   Add the chicken broth, fish sauce, lime juice, tamari sauce or coconut aminos, red curry paste, grated cinnamon, mushrooms, lemongrass, sea salt, and black pepper. Mix well. Close the pressure lid and cook on high mode for 5 minutes. When cooking time elapses, let the pressure to escape naturally for 5 minutes. Quick release the remaining pressure and open the lid. Add the coconut shrimp and milk. Stir to combine. Boil the soup on sauté mode for around 5 minutes. Let the soup rest for two minutes before serving. Serve with cilantro toppings.

Wild Salmon Tagine

INGREDIENTS (4 Servings)

Spice Paste:

41/2 oz of coriander leaves and stems

4 cloves of garlic

Juice from a lemon

Orange zest (one orange)

1 lemon zest

A tablespoon of ground paprika

1 tablespoon of apple cider vinegar

1 red chili (seeded and stem off)

A tablespoon of ground cumin

1/4 teaspoon of red pepper cayenne

1/4 teaspoon of sea salt

Tagine:

4 frozen salmon fillets

4 tablespoon of extra virgin organic olive oil

1 red onion

10 oz of sweet potatoes (peeled and diced)

2 carrots, diced

14 oz of chopped tomatoes (tinned)

A cup of stock, vegetable or fish

1.5 oz of dried cherries

2 oz of pitted olives

2 oranges (peeled and chopped)

DIRECTIONS (PREP + COOK TIME: 24 MINUTES) Preheat the Foodi pot. Puree all the spice paste ingredients. Spread a tablespoon of the paste on the fish. Melt butter in the Foodi and add the red onion, carrots, sweet potatoes, and the remaining spice mix. Sauté and stir for 5 minutes. Add the stock, tinned tomatoes, oranges, olives, and dried cherries. Place the frozen fish on top and seal the pressure lid. Cook on high mode for 4 minutes. Quick release the in-built vapor and open the lid. Serve your wild salmon tagine garnished with fresh herbs (preferably parsley and mint leaves.)

Gentle And Simple Fish

INGREDIENTS (4 Servings)

3 cups fish stock

1 onion, diced

1 cup broccoli, chopped

2 cups celery stalks, chopped

1 and ½ cups cauliflower, diced

1 carrot, sliced

1 pound white fish fillets, chopped

1 cup heavy cream 1 bay leaf

2 tablespoons butter

¼ teaspoon pepper

½ teaspoon salt

¼ teaspoon garlic powder

DIRECTIONS (PREP + COOK TIME: 25 MINUTES)

Set your Ninja Foodi to Saute mode and add butter, let it melt Add onion and carrots, cook for 3 minutes. Stir in remaining ingredients Lock lid and cook on HIGH pressure for 4 minutes.Naturally, release pressure over 10 minutes Discard bay leaf . Serve and enjoy!

Cool Shrimp Zoodles

INGREDIENTS (4 Servings)

4 cups zoodles

1 tablespoon basil, chopped

2 tablespoons Ghee

1 cup vegetable stock

2 garlic cloves, minced

2 tablespoons olive oil

½ lemon

½ teaspoon paprika

DIRECTIONS (PREP + COOK TIME: 8 MINUTES)

Set your Ninja Foodi to Saute mode and add ghee, let it heat up Add olive oil as well. Add garlic and cook for 1 minute Add lemon juice, shrimp and cook for 1 minute Stir in rest of the ingredients and lock lid, cook on LOW pressure for 5 minutes Quick release pressure and serve . Enjoy!

Awesome Cherry Tomato Mackerel

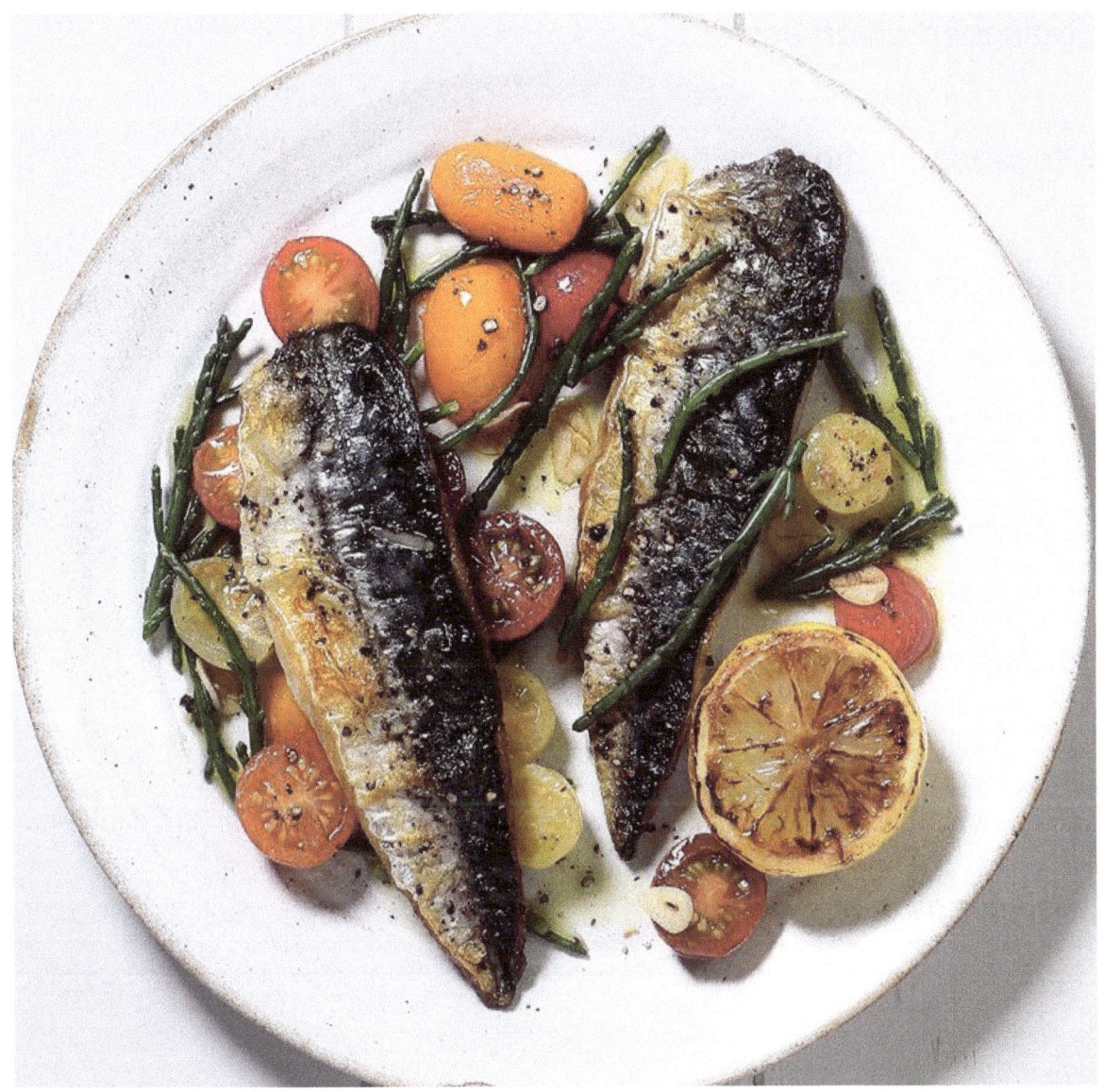

INGREDIENTS (4 Servings)

4 Mackerel fillets

¼ teaspoon onion powder

¼ teaspoon lemon powder

¼ teaspoon garlic powder

½ teaspoon salt

2 cups cherry tomatoes

3 tablespoons melted butter

1 and ½ cups of water

1 tablespoon black olives

DIRECTIONS (PREP + COOK TIME: 12 MINUTES)

Grease baking dish and arrange cherry tomatoes at the bottom of the dish Top with fillets sprinkle all spices. Drizzle melted butter over Add water to your Ninja Foodi Lower rack in Ninja Foodi and place baking dish on top of the rack Lock lid and cook on LOW pressure for 7 minutes . Quick release pressure. Serve and enjoy!

Packets Of Lemon And Dill Cod

INGREDIENTS (4 Servings)

2 tilapia cod fillets

Salt, pepper and garlic powder to taste

2 sprigs fresh dill

4 slices lemon

2 tablespoons butter

Layout 2 large squares of parchment paper

Place fillet in center of each parchment square and season with salt, pepper and garlic powder

On each fillet, place

1 sprig of dill,

2 lemon slices,

1 tablespoon butter

DIRECTIONS (PREP + COOK TIME: 10 MINUTES)

Place trivet at the bottom of your Ninja Foodi. Add 1 cup water into the pot Close parchment paper around fillets and fold to make a nice seal Place both packets in your pot . Lock lid and cook on HIGH pressure for 5 minutes Quick release pressure . Serve and enjoy!

Salmon Paprika

INGREDIENTS (4 Servings)

2 wild caught salmon fillets,

1 to 1 and ½ inches thick

2 teaspoons avocado oil

2 teaspoons paprika

Salt and pepper to taste

Green herbs to garnish

DIRECTIONS (PREP + COOK TIME: 12 MINUTES)

Season salmon fillets with salt, pepper, paprika, and olive oil Place
Crisping basket in your Ninja Foodi, and pre-heat your Ninja Foodie

at 390 degrees F Place insert insider your Foodi and place the fillet in the insert, lock Air Crisping lid and cook for 7 minutes. Once done, serve the fish with herbs on top. Enjoy!

Alaskan Cod Divine

INGREDIENTS (4 Servings)

1 large fillet, Alaskan Cod (Frozen)

1 cup cherry tomatoes

Salt and pepper to taste

Seasoning as you need

2 tablespoons butter

Olive oil as needed

DIRECTIONS (PREP + COOK TIME: 20 MINUTES)

Take an ovenproof dish small enough to fit inside your pot Add
tomatoes to the dish, cut large fish fillet into 2-3 serving pieces

and lay them on top of tomatoes. Season with salt, pepper, and your seasoning Top each fillet with 1 tablespoon butter and drizzle olive oil Add 1 cup of water to the pot.Place trivet to the Ninja Foodi and place dish on the trivet Lock lid and cook on HIGH pressure for 9 minutes.Release pressure naturally over 10 minutes Serve and enjoy!

Lemon And Pepper Salmon Delight

INGREDIENTS (4 Servings)

¾ cup of water

Sprigs of parsley, basil, tarragon

1 pound salmon, skin on   3 teaspoons ghee

¾ teaspoon salt

½ teaspoon pepper

½ lemon, sliced

1 red bell pepper, julienned

1 carrot, julienned

DIRECTIONS (PREP + COOK TIME: 10 MINUTES)

Set your Ninja Foodi to Saute mode and add water and herbs Place a steamer rack and add the salmon. Drizzle ghee on top of the salmon Season with pepper and salt. Cover lemon slices on top Lock up the lid and cook on HIGH pressure for 3 minutes Release the pressure naturally over 10 minutes Transfer the salmon to a platter. Add veggies to your pot and set the pot to Saute mode Cook for 1-2 minutes. Serve the cooked vegetables with salmon. Enjoy!

Delightful Salmon Fillets

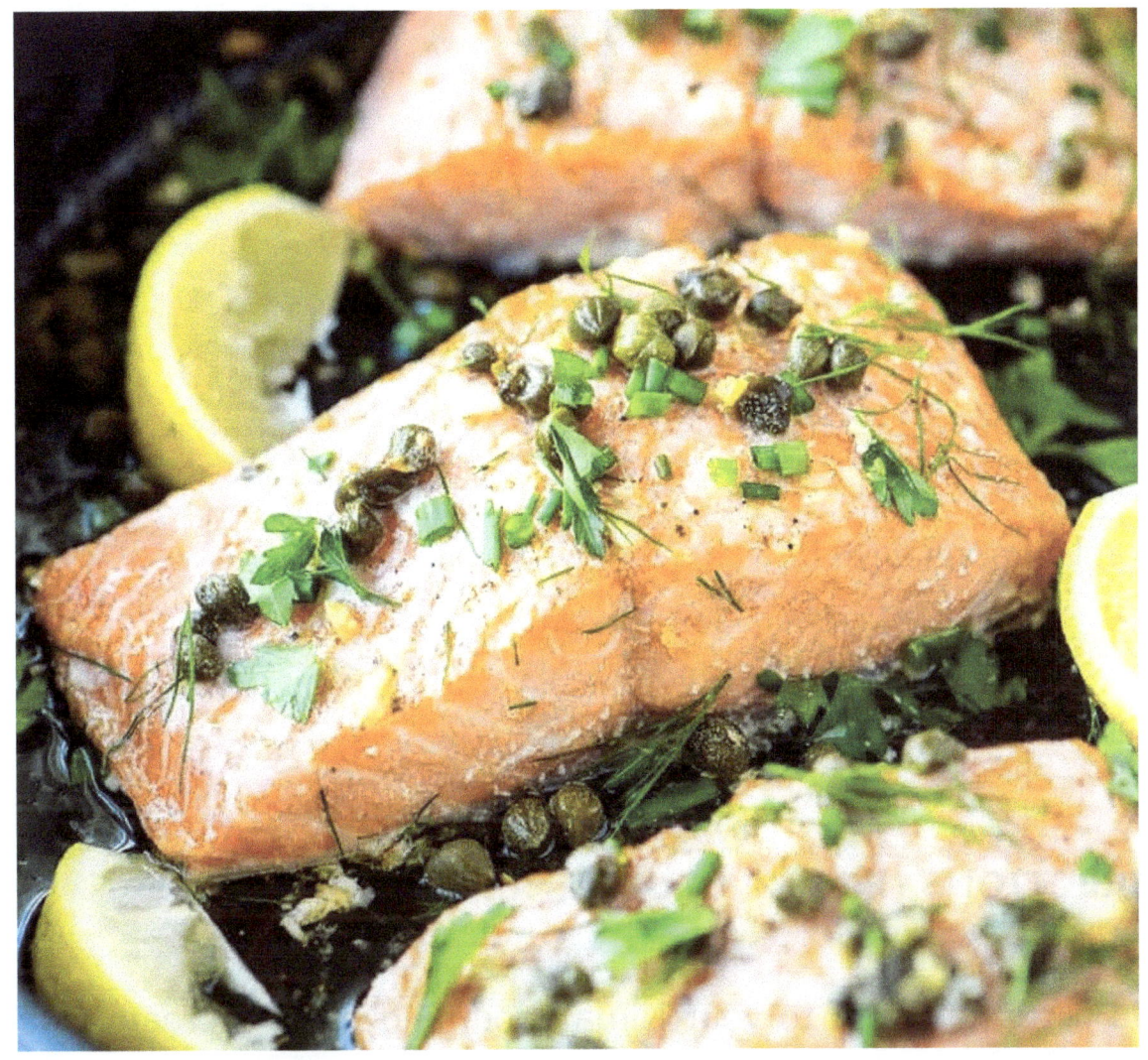

INGREDIENTS (4 Servings)

2 salmon fillets

¼ cup onion, chopped

2 stalks green onion stalks, chopped

1 whole egg

Almond meal as needed

Salt and pepper to taste

2 tablespoons olive oil

DIRECTIONS (PREP + COOK TIME: 10 MINUTES)

Add a cup of water to your Ninja Foodi and place a steamer rack on top Place the fish. Season the fish with salt and pepper and lock up the lid Cook on HIGH pressure for 3 minutes. Once done, quick release the pressure Remove the fish and allow it to cool Break the fillets into a bowl and add egg, yellow and green onions Add ½ a cup of almond meal and mix with your hand. Divide the mixture into patties Take a large skillet and place it over medium heat. Add oil and cook the patties.Enjoy!

Cucumber And Salmon Mix

INGREDIENTS (4 Servings)

1 pound salmon steaks

½ cup plain low-fat Greek yogurt

½ cup cucumber, peeled and diced

1 tablespoon fresh dill, chopped

1 tablespoon olive oil

½ teaspoon ground coriander

1 teaspoon fresh lemon juice

1 cup of water

Salt and pepper to taste

DIRECTIONS (PREP + COOK TIME: 10 MINUTES)

Mix in low-fat Greek yogurt, dill, cucumber, a pinch of salt and pepper each, mix well and put in the fridge Brush salmon steaks with olive oil, season salmon with salt, pepper and coriander and lemon juice. Add water to Ninja Foodi and place a steamer rack Add fish fillets on rack and lock lid. Cook on HIGH pressure for 3 minutes Release pressure naturally over 10 minutes . Open the lid and serve salmon with cucumber sauce. Enjoy!

Tilapia And Asparagus Delight

INGREDIENTS (4 Servings)

1 bunch asparagus

4-6 tilapia fillets

8-12 tablespoons lemon juice

Pepper for seasoning

Lemon juice for seasoning

½ tablespoons for clarified butter, for each fillet

DIRECTIONS (PREP + COOK TIME: 2 hours and 10 MINUTES)

Cut single pieces of foil for the fillets Divide the bundle of asparagus into even number depending on the number of your fillets Lay the fillets on each of the pieces of foil and sprinkle pepper and add a teaspoon of lemon juice. Add clarified butter and top with asparagus Fold the foil over the fish and seal the ends.Repeat with all the fillets and transfer to Ninja Foodi Cook on SLOW COOK MODE (HIGH) for 2 hours. Enjoy!

The Great Poached Salmon

INGREDIENTS (4 Servings)

16-ounce salmon fillet, skin on

4 scallions, chopped Zest of 1 lemon

½ a teaspoon of fennel seeds

1 teaspoon white wine vinegar

1 bay leaf

½ cup dry white wine

2 cups chicken broth

¼ cup fresh dill

Salt and pepper

DIRECTIONS (PREP + COOK TIME: 15 MINUTES)

Add the listed ingredients to your Ninja Foodi, stir well Lock lid and cook on HIGH pressure for 4 minutes. Release pressure naturally over 10 minutes Serve and enjoy!

Garlic Sauce And Mussels

INGREDIENTS (4 Servings)

3 pounds mussels

1 tablespoon extra-virgin olive oil

4 garlic cloves, minced

1 large roasted bell pepper

¾ cup fish stock

½ cup white wine vinegar

1/8 teaspoon red pepper flakes

2 tablespoons cashew cream

3 tablespoons parsley, chopped

DIRECTIONS (PREP + COOK TIME: 16 MINUTES)

Clean the mussels well and scrub them, debeard if needed. Make a steaming liquid Set your Ninja Foodi to Saute mode and add olive oil, allow it to heat up Add garlic and cook for 1 minute Add roasted red pepper, vinegar, fish stock, red pepper flakes and stir Add mussels to the Ninja Foodi and lock up the lid Cook on HIGH pressure for 1 minute and quick release the pressure Remove the lid and check the mussels, if they are open then enjoy If not, lock up the lid and steam for 1 minute more. Garnish with a bit of parsley. Enjoy!

Medi-Bass Stew

INGREDIENTS (6 Servings)

1 pound sea bass fillets, patted dry and cut into

2 inch chunks

3 tablespoons Cajun seasoning, divided

½ teaspoon salt

2 tablespoons extra virgin olive oil

2 yellow onion, diced

2 bell peppers, diced

4 celery stalks, diced

1 can (28 ounces) diced tomatoes, drained

¼ cup tomato paste

1 and ½ cups veggie broth

2 pounds large shrimp, peeled and deveined

DIRECTIONS (PREP + COOK TIME: 28 MINUTES) Set your Pot to Saute mode at a temperature of Medium-HIGH heat, let it pre-heat for 5 minutes Season sea bass on both sides with 1 and ½ tablespoons Cajun seasoning and ¼ teaspoon salt. Put 1 tablespoon oil and sea bass in your pre-heated pot. Saute for 4 minutes Add remaining 1 tablespoon oil and onions to the pot and cook for 3 minutes, add bell peppers, celery, and 1 and ½ tablespoons Cajun seasoning to the pot. Cook for 2 minutes more Add sea bass, diced tomatoes, tomato paste, broth to the pot, place the lid and seal the valves Cook on HIGH pressure for 5 minutes, quick release the pressure once did Set your pot to Saute mode again with the temperature set at Medium-HIGH mode and add shrimp. Place lid and seal the pressure valve, cook for 4 minutes until the shrimp is opaque Season with ¼ teaspoon salt and serve, enjoy!

Salmon in Dill Sauce

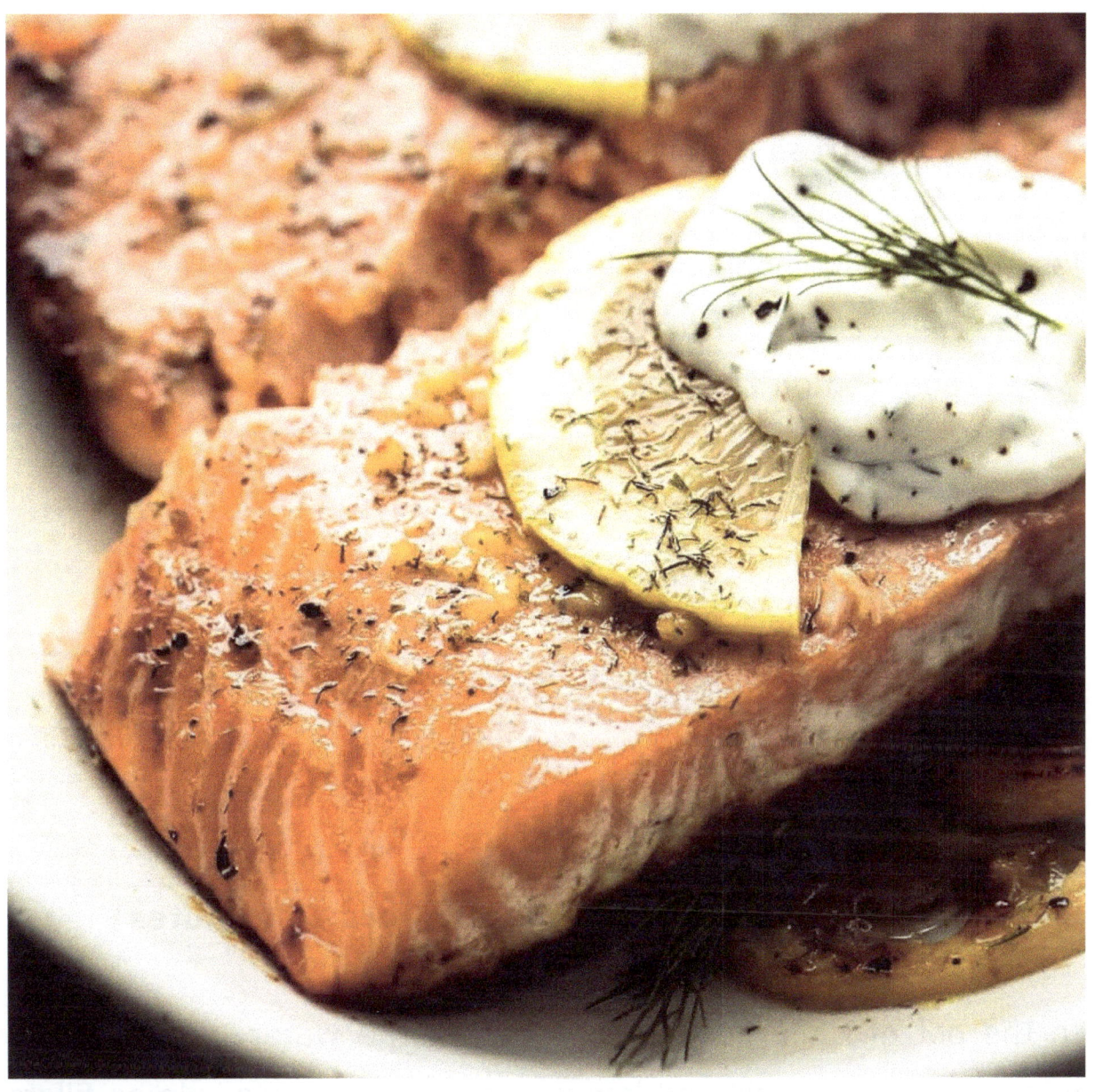

INGREDIENTS (6 Servings)

2 cups water

1 cup chicken broth

2 tablespoons fresh lemon juice

¼ cup fresh dill, chopped

½ teaspoon lemon zest, grated

6 (4-ounce) salmon fillets

Salt and ground black pepper, as required

DIRECTIONS (Prep + Cook Time: 2 hours 10 minutes)

In the pot of Ninja Foodi, mix together the water, broth, lemon juice, lemon juice, dill and lemon zest. Arrange the salmon fillets on top, skin side down and sprinkle with salt and black pepper. Close the Ninja Foodi with crisping lid and select "Slow Cooker". Set on "Low" for 1-2 hours. Press "Start/Stop" to begin cooking. Open the lid and serve hot.

Spicy Catfish

INGREDIENTS (2 Servings)

2 tablespoons almond flour

1 teaspoon red chili powder

½ teaspoon paprika

½ teaspoon garlic powder

Salt, as required

2 (6-ounces) catfish fillets

1 tablespoon olive oil

DIRECTIONS (Prep + Cook Time: 23 minutes)

Arrange the greased "Cook & Crisp Basket" in the pot of Ninja Foodi. Close the Ninja Foodi with crisping lid and select "Air Crisp". Set the temperature to 400 degrees F for 5 minutes. Press "Start/Stop" to begin preheating. In a bowl, mix together the flour, paprika, garlic powder and salt. Add the catfish fillets and coat with the mixture evenly. Now, coat each fillet with oil. After preheating, open the lid. Place the catfish fillets into the "Cook & Crisp Basket". Close the Ninja Foodi with crisping lid and select "Air Crisp". Set the temperature to 400 degrees F for 13 minutes. Press "Start/Stop" to begin cooking. Flip the fish fillets once halfway through. Open the lid and serve hot.

Cod Parcel

INGREDIENTS (2 Servings)

2 (4-ounce) cod fillets

½ teaspoon garlic powder

Salt and ground black pepper, as required

2 fresh dill sprigs

4 lemon slices

2 tablespoons butter

DIRECTIONS (Prep + Cook Time: 23 minutes)

Arrange 2 large parchment squares onto a smooth surface. Place 1 fillet in the center of each parchment square and sprinkle with garlic powder, salt and black pepper. Top each fillet with 1 dill sprig, 2 lemon slices and 1 tablespoon of butter. Fold each parchment paper around the fillets to seal. In the pot of Ninja Foodi, place 1 cup of water. Arrange the "Reversible Rack" in the pot of Ninja Foodi. Place the fish parcels over the "Reversible Rack". Close the Ninja Foodi with the pressure lid and place the pressure valve to "Seal" position. Select "Pressure" and set to "High for 8 minutes. Press "Start/Stop" to begin cooking. Switch the valve to "Vent" and do a "Quick" release. Open the lid and transfer the fish parcels onto serving plates. Carefully unwrap the parcels and serve.

Scallops with Spinach

INGREDIENTS (3 Servings)

1 (10-ounce) package frozen spinach, thawed and drained

12 sea scallops Olive oil cooking spray

Salt and ground black pepper, as required

¾ cup heavy whipping cream

1 tablespoon tomato paste

1 teaspoon garlic, minced

1 tablespoon fresh basil, chopped

DIRECTIONS (Prep + Cook Time: 25 minutes) Arrange the greased "Cook & Crisp Basket" in the pot of Ninja Foodi. Close the

Ninja Foodi with crisping lid and select "Air Crisp". Set the temperature to 350 degrees F for 5 minutes. Press "Start/Stop" to begin preheating. In the bottom of a 7-inch heatproof pan, place the spinach. Spray each scallop with cooking spray and then sprinkle with a little salt and black pepper. Arrange scallops on top of the spinach in a single layer. In a bowl, add the cream, tomato paste, garlic, basil, salt and black pepper and mix well. Place the cream mixture over the spinach and scallops evenly. After preheating, open the lid. Place the pan into "Cook & Crisp Basket". Close the Ninja Foodi with crisping lid and select "Air Crisp". Set the temperature to 350 degrees F for 10 minutes. Press "Start/Stop" to begin cooking. Open the lid and serve hot.

Buttered Crab Legs

INGREDIENTS (2 Servings)

1½ pounds frozen crab legs

Salt, as required

2 tablespoons butter, melted

DIRECTIONS (Prep + Cook Time: 19 minutes) In the pot of Ninja Foodi, place 1 cup of water and 1 teaspoon of salt. Arrange the "Reversible Rack" in the pot of Ninja Foodi. Place the crab legs over the "Reversible Rack "and sprinkle with salt. Close the Ninja Foodi with the pressure lid and place the pressure valve to "Seal" position. Select "Pressure" and set to "High" for 4 minutes. Press "Start/Stop" to begin cooking. Switch the valve to "Vent" and do a "Quick" release. Open the lid and transfer crab legs onto a serving platter. Drizzle with butter and serve.

Creamy Shrimp Scampi

INGREDIENTS (6 Servings)

2 tablespoons of butter

1lb of shrimp, frozen

4 garlic cloves, minced

1/4 teaspoons of red pepper flakes

1/2 teaspoon of paprika

2 cups of uncooked low-carbohydrate pasta (Carbanada)

1 cup of chicken broth

1/2 cup of half and half

1/2 cup of mozzarella cheese

Pepper

DIRECTIONS (PREP + COOK TIME: 15 MINUTES) Melt butter on sauté mode. Add the red pepper flakes and garlic and cook until the garlic browns. Add the paprika, frozen shrimp, pepper, and the noodles. Add the chicken broth and close the pressure lid. Cook for 2 minutes and quick release the in-built pressure. Set your Foodi to sauté mode and add the cheese. Add the half and half and stir. Cook the mixture until everything melt. Close the crisping lid and bake at 350°F or until the internal temperature drops to 165° F. Allow it to cool before serving.

Keto Clam Chowder

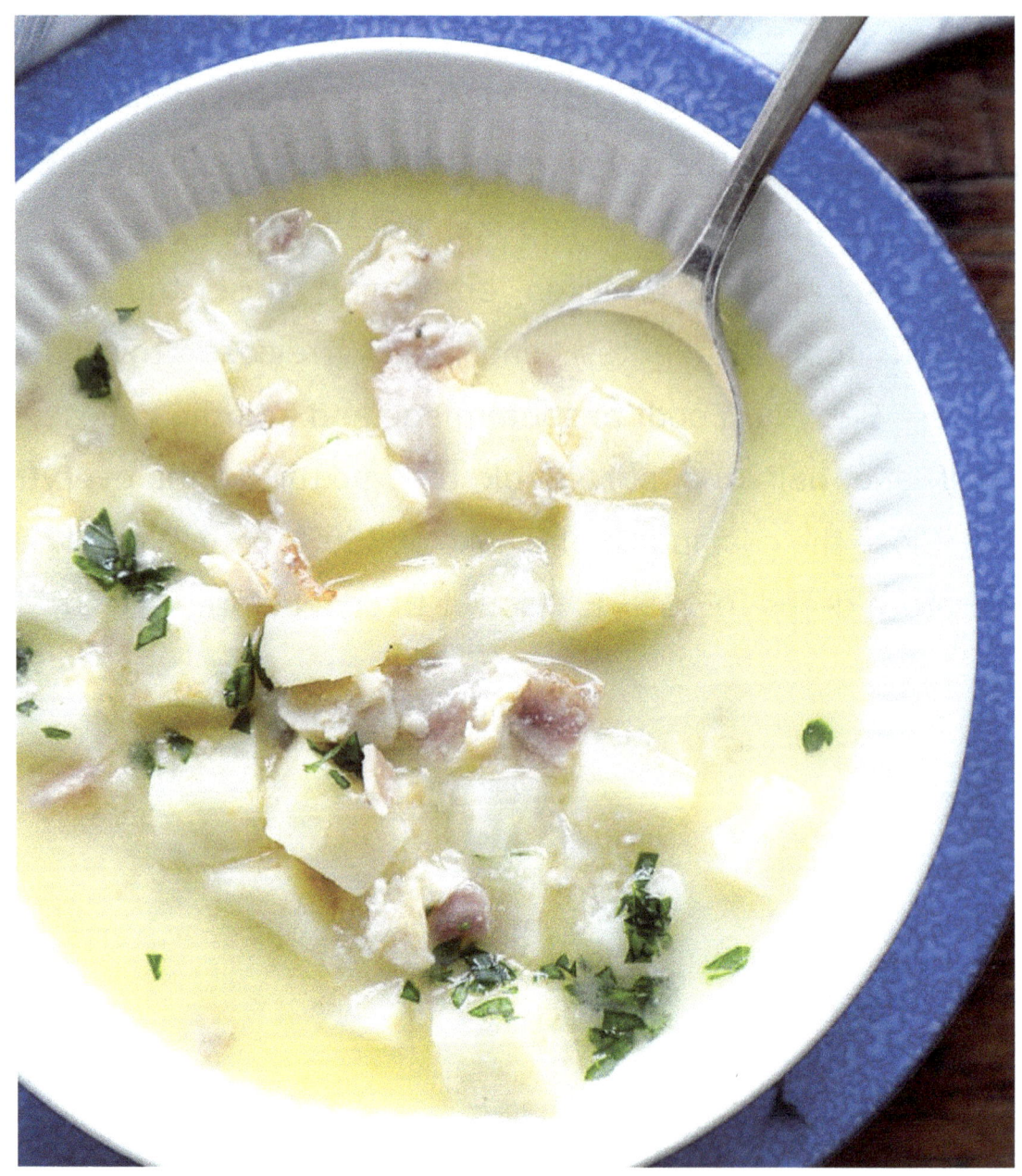

INGREDIENTS (6 Servings)

4 slices (4.2 oz) of bacon, chopped

4 tablespoons of unsalted butter

1 white onion, diced

2 celery stalks, diced

2 garlic cloves, minced

3 cups of diced turnips

1 teaspoon of sea salt

Few sprigs of fresh thyme

1/4 teaspoon of black pepper

A cup of clam juice 1 lb of clams Optional

1/4 teaspoon of cayenne

2 (10 oz) cans of baby clams, boiled (reserve juice)

1 1/2 glasses of heavy cream

DIRECTIONS (PREP + COOK TIME: 25 MINUTES) Preheat your Foodi on sauté mode for a minute. Add the bacon and butter and allow it to fry for 5 minutes or until its crispy. Add onions, celery, garlic, and spices. Sauté for another 3 minutes or until the spices tenderize. Add the diced turnips and clam juice. Close the pressure lid and cook on low mode for a minute. Once cooked quick release the pressure and open the lid carefully. Add your littleneck clams and cream. Stir. Sauté the mixture on high mode for 4 minutes. Mash half of the turnips using a tomato masher. Let the turnips simmer for 5- 7 minutes while stirring frequently. Serve your Keto clam chowder while garnished with thyme.

Conclusion

Did you appreciate trying these brand-new and also scrumptious recipes?

Unfortunately we have actually come to the end of this recipe book pertaining to the use of the fantastic Ninja Foodi multi-cooker, which I truly wish you taken pleasure in.

To improve your health we want to advise you to integrate physical activity and also a vibrant way of life along with following these superb recipes, so regarding highlight the renovations. we will be back soon with an increasing number of appealing vegetarian recipes, a large hug, see you soon.

9 781667 108452